Published by: Rebecca Lowe dba Manual Therapy of Nashville

Model: Lori Winter

Editors: Lori Winter, Edith Liechty

Text, Illustrations, & Cover Design: Drew Winter, edited by Preston Kincaid

Portrait: David Molnar

Cover & Cube Photos by: Darien Photography

ISBN: 9798720660444

Rebecca Lowe

THE omPT CUBE:
Self-Care with the omPT Cube

The omPT Cube

REBECCA LOWE

Contents

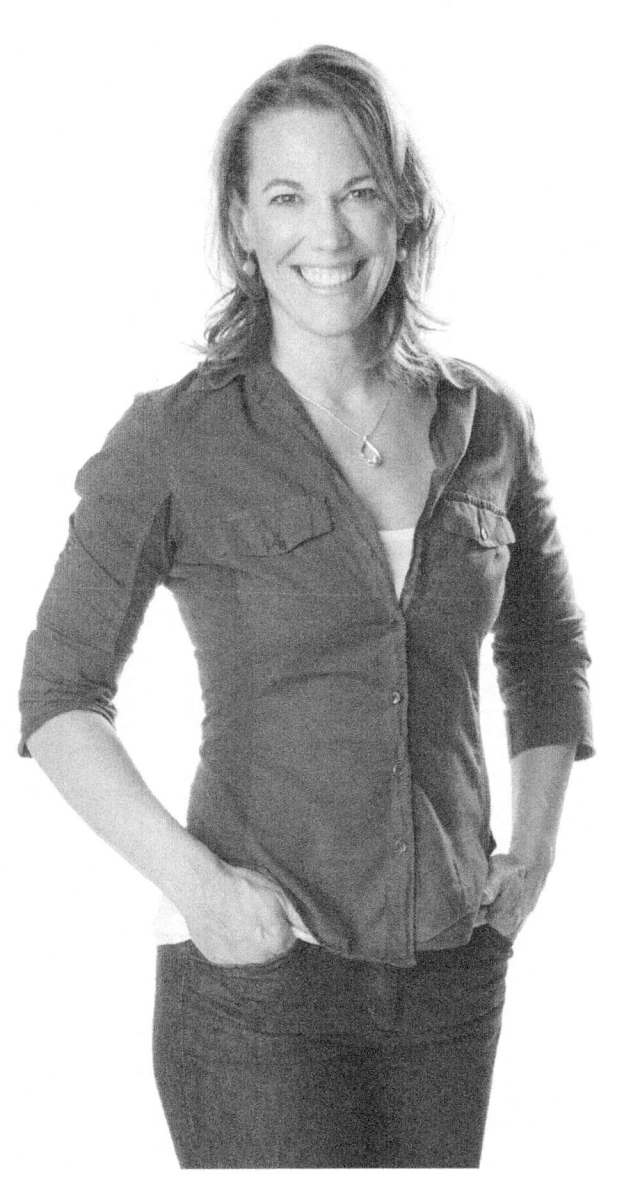

Background

Rebecca Lowe developed the omPT Cube and other products when she realized that her clients would get better, but often they could not stay better. Life happens and muscles and bones do not usually stay in place without someone doing something for their own care and maintenance.

She developed the omPT Cube and started teaching her clients how to treat themselves, even their own spine issues. Besides self-treatment, people need movement and strength to stay at their optimum body functioning. So, omPT Cube is best when used alongside a yoga practice, or other regular routine of fitness and movement.

Rebecca Lowe, who has over 26 years of experience and study in the specialty of Orthopedic Manual Physical Therapy (OMPT), developed the omPT Cube and other products to help therapists and clientstake an important role in their own care.

It is Rebecca's mission to empower others to connect to their whole person - body, mind, heart, and spirit - to help them transform their lives and live in freedom. She has found that she can inspire people and teach these tools. She has heard gratitude from many, many clients and students in classes that the Cube has given them power over their own pain and tightness. The omPT Cube has been taken around the world in backpacks on mountain treks and in cars and carry-ons and purses. Once you learn how to treat yourself, you will always know how to treat yourself.

This is her offering to help heal the world, but it cannot be accomplished alone. To do this, we need everyone doing their part to bring this about, each person taking care of themselves. In addition to being an OMPT, Rebecca is also an author, educator, private practice owner (Manual Therapy of Nashville, LLC), registered yoga teacher, consultant, and mentor. She is passionate about empowering people to heal. She is sharing this combination of specific movement and global movements in yoga and PT as one of the best ways to treat ourselves and stay better. Let's be free.

"I wake up most mornings feeling stiff or sore."

"I sit all day at work, and my hips and low back are paying the price."

"Lots of driving and computer work mean my posture could use improvement."

"I carry tension in my shoulders and neck."

Do any of those ailments describe you? Have you thought these issues were simply a normal part of modern life? You're definitely not alone. I meet with patients in my practice almost every day who fit this profile. But while these ailments are certainly common, they don't have to be your normal!

It's my mission in life to empower as many people as possible to connect to their whole person - body, mind, heart, and spirit - to help them transform their lives and live in freedom.

As an Orthopedic Manual Physical Therapist, I created the omPT Cube to give clients and practitioners a tool to treat their own body, even very specifically the spine.

Over my 26+ years of experience and study, I've seen many, many people improve and get better when they would come see me in my clinic. But, in order to stay better, they often required some type of maintenance. Life happens, and muscles and bones do not stay in place without some type of consistent care and maintenance program. In addition to this self-treatment, people also need movement and strength to stay at an optimal level of body functioning. So, the omPT Cube is best when used in the context of a wellness routine that includes good nutrition and some form of exercise. As a Physical Therapist, I want my patients to get better and stay better.

I applaud you for taking this first step toward feeling and functioning better. By purchasing this omPT Cube you're taking positive action for your health. I want to encourage you that there is hope! I'm a firm believer in holding on to hope, even in the midst of pain — so much so that I wrote a book* about it.

Let's begin!

* *Restoring Hope in Chronic Pain: A Whole-Person Perspective From an Orthopedic Manual Physical Therapist (OMPT)* is available on Amazon.com

How will I know if the omPT Cube is right for me?

I developed the omPT Cube for those people who are able to participate in wellness classes — fitness, movement, yoga, etc. As long as your ailments fall into the categories of minor range of motion limitations or minimal discomfort and tightness, then the omPT Cube is absolutely worth trying. You'll learn how to treat your own body in ways that are similar to and supportive of treatments from a Physical Therapist or other bodyworker.

"Normal" discomfort and tightness would be described as:

1. Feeling moderate pain or discomfort (a 6 out of 10 on the pain scale). Anything more than this is most likely a more severe or significant problem that would require a professional evaluation.

2. You do not have referred pain to other areas, or it is minimal. This means the pain stays in one place and does not travel to other areas. You should not have any lines of pain, particularly if it is sharp, shooting, electrical, or burning. All pain is not the same, and you want to use the omPT Cube if you have more "typical" musculoskeletal issues.

3. You feel pain with movement, but not at rest. This is one indicator of mechanical pain (the kind of ailments that the omPT Cube is best suited to address). If you move something, and you can make it better or worse, then more than likely it is related to a joint or muscle. If you have constant pain, it may still be a mechanical problem, but it may be inflamed, which means it needs rest and not movement at this stage. Or, it could indicate something more serious.

4. You are still able to participate in daily recreational and fitness activities. You may feel pain or mild discomfort or tightness while doing it, but it does not prevent you from doing it. If you have to stop what you're doing, or you can't do it at all, because of the discomfort, you'll want to have a professional evaluate the problem before continuing or starting any movement or exercise program or using the OMPT Cube.

5. You do not have pain that wakes you up at night. Pain that wakes you up at night is a more significant problem. It may still be a muscle or joint issue, but it could also be something more serious. Also, if you aren't sleeping well, that needs to be addressed first. We heal when we sleep.

6. You do not have significant weakness or neurological deficits. Neurological problems are neurological in origin and using omPT Cube wouldn't be appropriate to address the root of

the issue in that case. The problem in the nerve may or may not be related to a muscle or bone tissue. Numbness, tingling, and burning are all signs that a nerve is involved.

If the descriptions above apply to you, congratulations! I believe omPT Cube can be an integral part of your healing process. You will benefit from the exercises described in this book using the omPT Cube.

But, safety is a primary concern. Most importantly, you don't want to risk making an issue worse than it is. The omPT Cube is not appropriate for you if you experience:

• A high level of pain

• Unusual or neurological symptoms

• Inability to perform normal daily activities

In any of these cases, do not try the omPT Cube until you can get your problem evaluated by a healthcare professional.

The following are other, more specific reasons not to use the omPT Cube. This is not an exhaustive list by any means:

• Anyone with unexplained or undiagnosed pain

• Signs of infection or inflammation: swelling, heat

• Acute or recent injury

• Non-musculoskeletal pain

• Those who do not have intact sensation on their skin

• Neurological disorders and neuromas

- Severe or inflammatory arthritis such as ankylosing spondylosis, rheumatoid arthritis, traumatic arthritis

- Spondylolisthesis – at the same and nearby spinal levels

- Osteoporosis, osteopenia

- Peripheral vascular disease

- Arteriosclerosis

- Deep vein thrombosis (DVT)

- Skin – sores/wounds/infection

- Infectious disease i.e. pink eye, colds, contagious illness

With the following specific injuries and illnesses, you would want to use the omPT Cube with caution and observe if the omPT Cube affects your condition. This is not an exhaustive list:

- Body unawareness

- Hypermobility syndromes and collagen disorders

- Arthritis

- Migraines vs headaches

- Chronic regional pain syndrome or fibromyalgia

- Cardiovascular disease

- Respiratory disease

- Psychological disorders

There are two other reasons you would want to consult a professional when using the omPT Cube:

1. You started the omPT Cube, but experienced a moderate or significant adverse response.

2. The omPT Cube seems to be helping your condition, but it appears you could improve more effectively with the addition of specific assessment and treatment. Perhaps you have plateaued in your improvement, or the location of symptoms may indicate altered joint mechanics or a problem with stability.

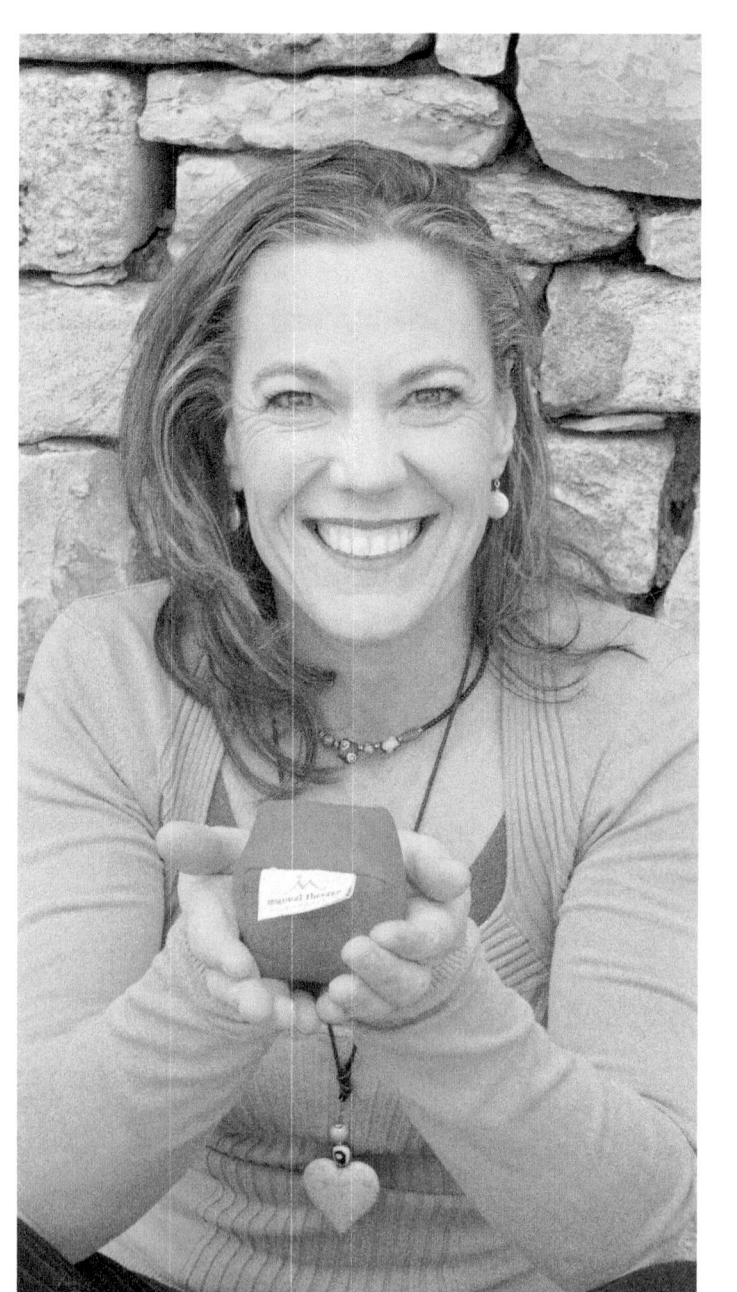

The omPT Cube

This is the omPT Cube; it's simple. It's not a technical gadget with buttons and levers. No assembly required!

Even though it's simple, it has the potential to be a powerful tool to treat your body. I'm excited to show you how to use it effectively.

The omPT Cube is portable and can be used almost anywhere. Toss it in your gym bag, your purse, or your carry-on bag on an airplane. Some people even buy extras — one at work and one at home.

The canvas fabric can be spot cleaned with warm water and mild soap, but shouldn't be immersed in water. If you're worried about keeping it clean, you can always keep it in the plastic bag it arrived in. It will work just the same!

I've chosen a manufacturer that I trust to craft the omPT Cubes with exceptional quality. It should be able to withstand your full body weight when standing on it, up to about 180 pounds, though above that, you can simply avoid putting your entire bodyweight on the omPT Cube when treating the feet. Treating other areas of the body should be fine for almost anyone. If your omPT Cube does break within the first 30 days of purchasing, please contact us and we will happily replace it free of charge.

A word of caution — if you have pets, you may want to avoid leaving the omPT Cube on the floor unattended. They look very similar to balls or chew toys and Rover won't know the difference! Unfortunately, we can't replace your omPT Cube if the dog ate your homework. ;-)

The Whole Person

We are whole people. Our body, mind, heart, and spirit are all connected. The most effective way to treat your whole person is to address not only the physical body, but also your emotions, your mind, and your spirit.

The omPT Cube is not the end-all-be-all program for health and healing. No one program or tool possibly can be. But I'm confident that the omPT Cube can be an extremely powerful part of your healing journey, especially when combined with other approaches like a nutrient-rich diet, deep breathing practices, positive affirmations, and inner emotional work or counseling.

I also love how the omPT Cube integrates and overlaps with other healing modalities like reflexology, acupressure, and myofascial release. You'll see notes throughout this book regarding the connections.

Using the omPT Cube

The basic foundational principle for the omPT Cube is getting your bodyweight over the omPT Cube anywhere there's muscle. We want to use the omPT Cube on muscle, not bone. If you feel like you're on a bone, you probably are. Simply adjust the placementand try again.

We'll be massaging the muscle to release areas of tension, and, in some cases, to move the bones in the surrounding area.

Knots in the muscles all have different causes, but are known as trigger points. Research has shown that trigger points are areas of muscle fibers which, due to increased contraction, have altered mechanical, electrical, vascular, and chemical properties. Many of these trigger points can be reduced or eliminated by the mechanical stimulation and pressure from the omPT Cube.

When you're using the omPT Cube on these tight, sore, or tender areas, think about 360 degree movement. Shift your body weight slightly side to side. Turn or rotate over the omPT Cube.

Don't be afraid to explore different positions and discover therapeutic sensations that arise. You can trust your body to tell youwhat it needs. Learn to listen to what your body is telling you. It'salways talking!

Sometimes breathing is all the movement you'll want in a certain area. The expansion of your torso as you inhale will provide excellent movement of the body against the omPT Cube.

We also want to know the difference between pain and therapeutic sensations. Think 'ooo, that feels kind of good,' not 'ow!'

Breathing

Breathing is key when using the omPT Cube. Above all, just don't hold your breath!

Many of us aren't breathing as fully as we should be. Our breath is incredibly important to the overall function of our bodies. It oxygenates our blood, regulates our nervous system, and helps to clear our mind — just to name a few.

There are many different breath work techniques and deep breathing practices. Feel free to choose the one(s) you prefer. I'll include a couple of my favorites here. These can be incorporated with your omPT Cube work or performed on their own at any time.

Both of these breathing practices can re-set the autonomic nervous system and help it return to parasympathetic activity (non-fight or flight or freeze mode), allowing it to heal. Make sure your belly is "soft" and expands on the inhale. It will allow more relaxation, compassion, and self-acceptance versus power and control. Let yourself really relax.

Box Breathing

Imagine a box with equidistant sides. Starting from the bottom corner, inhale on a count of 4, then pause at the top of the breath for a count of 4. Exhale slowly and intentionally on a count of 4, then pause at the bottom of the breath for a count of 4. You've returned to the starting position, where you can begin again.

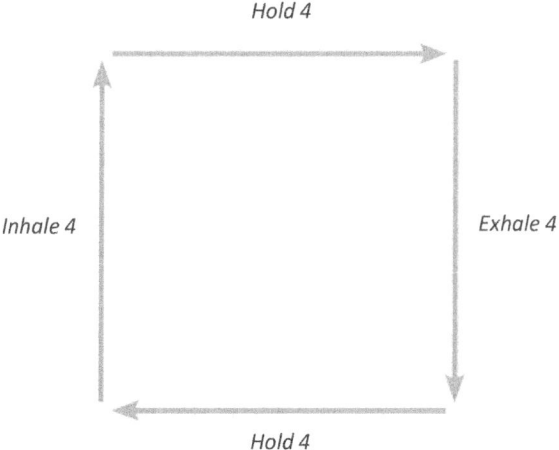

Hold 4

Inhale 4

Exhale 4

Hold 4

6-4-8 Breathing

In this technique, you'll be inhaling on a count of 6, holding the breath for a count of 4, then exhaling thoroughly on a count of 8. You can even cough or laugh at the bottom of the exhale to expel all the air from your lungs.

The pace of your counting doesn't matter, as long as the ratios of 6-4-8 are consistent. Aim for ten repetitions at least 3 times per day. If you find you become a little light-headed, try a quicker pace or take periodic rests before beginning again.

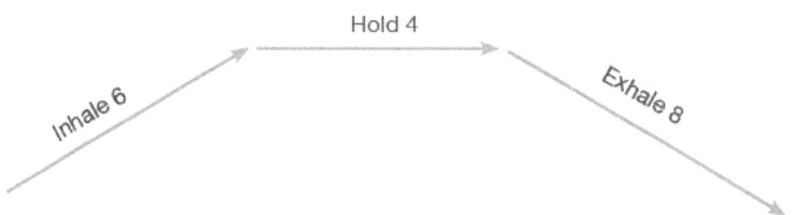

The Techniques

Here, we'll take an in-depth look at each area of the body and talk about how to use the omPT Cube there.

> **NOTE**
>
> The Tests and Re-tests included here aren't necessary every time you use your omPT Cube, but they are a great way to become more aware of your body day to day and to see almost right away if using the omPT Cube is positively affecting an area of your body.

Lower Legs

Test: Standing, place hands on wall or other support for balance. Take one leg back, first with knee straight, then with knee bent. Look and feel for any calf or ankle tightness.

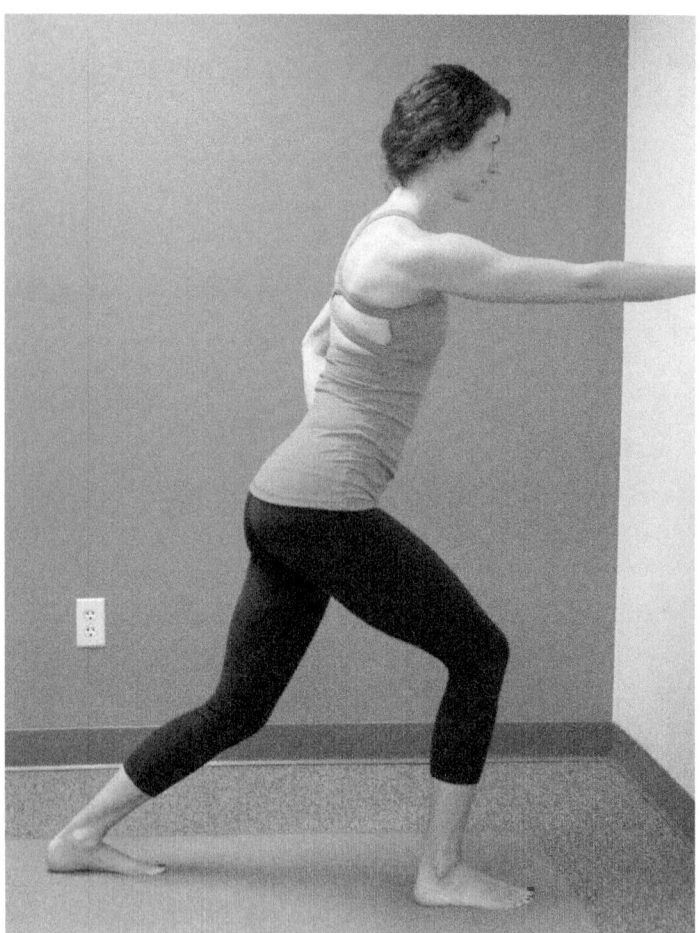

Treat: Feet.

Place one foot on the omPT Cube and begin to add pressure. Imagine two rays on the bottom of your feet, one on the inside and one on the outside. Work your way up each ray starting from the heel, finding areas to loosen, massage, and treat. Finish with the omPT Cube in the center of your forefoot, feeling the toes splay apart.

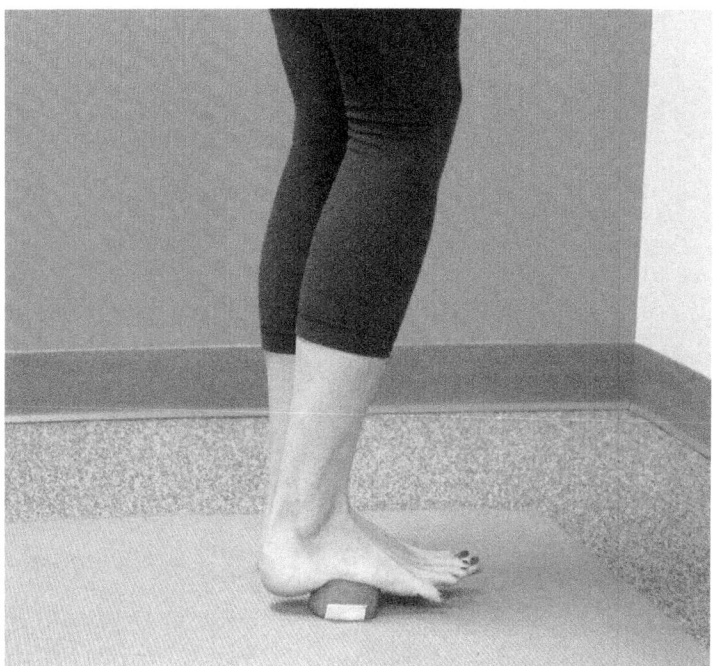

FUN FACT

In the practice of Reflexology, every part of the body is represented on the soles of the feet (as well as the hands and ears). It follows that using the omPT Cube on the feet can positively influence the entire body!

Test: Sit on your heels, first with the tops of the feet flat on the floor, then with the toes tucked under. Look and feel for ankle and anterior tibialis muscle tightness.

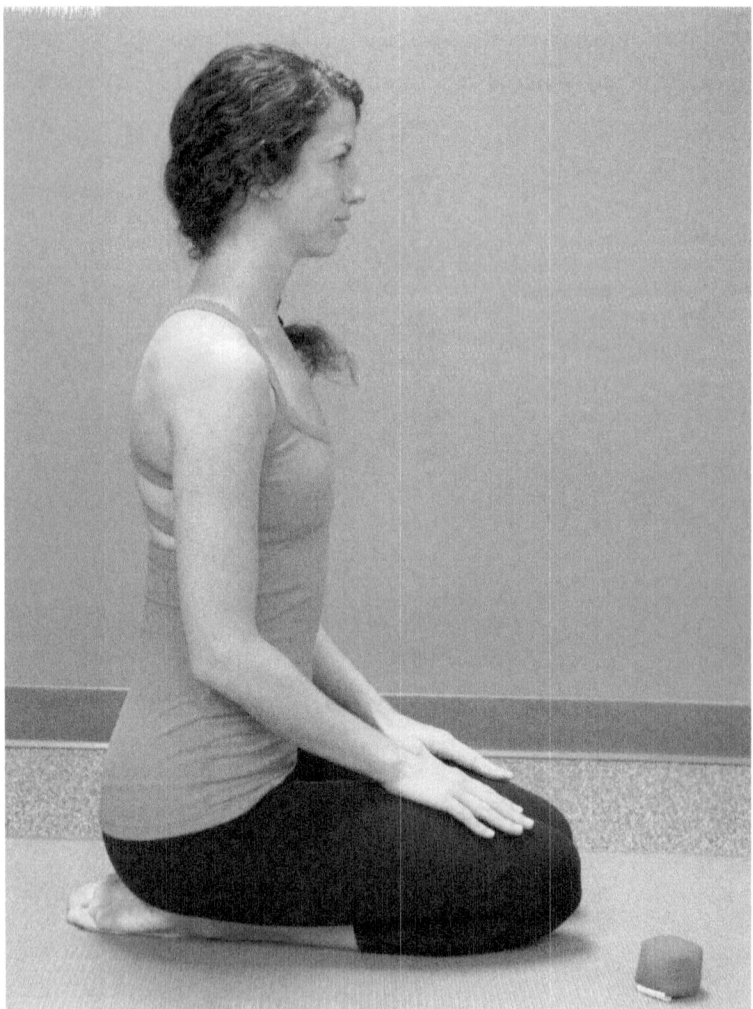

Treat: Anterior Tibialis (the muscle next to the shin bone).

Place the omPT Cube under the shin along the outside of the shin bone. You may need to lean to the side slightly to get the weight of your body over the omPT Cube effectively.

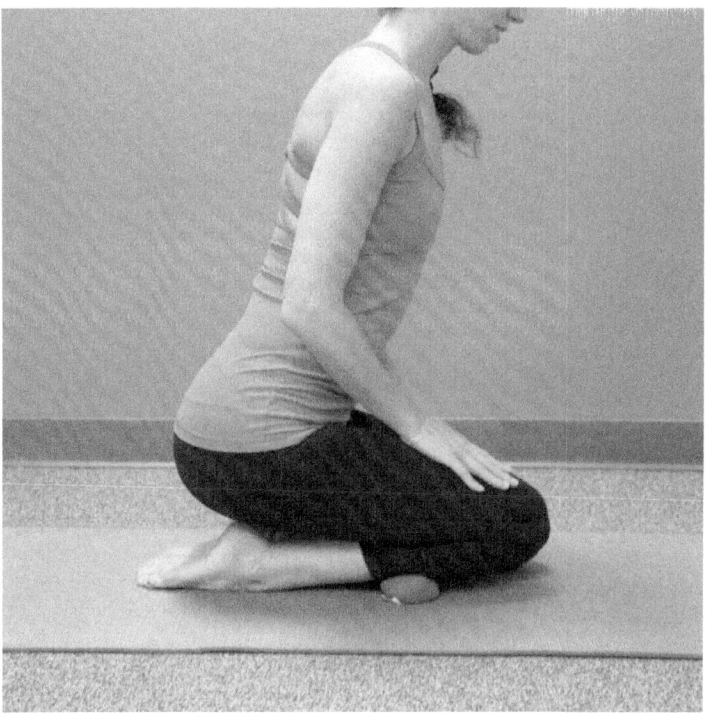

FUN FACT

In Traditional Chinese Medicine, the acupressure point Stomach 36 is located on the front of the leg, one hand width (four fingers) below the kneecap, on the outside, in the depression between the shin bone and the leg muscle. It's one of the most widely used acupressure and acupuncture points and is indicated to help with stress, fatigue, irritability, anxiety, allergies, gastrointestinal discomfort, nausea, vomiting, reproductive system disorders, and more.

Treat: Calves and hamstrings.

Sitting on your heels, place the omPT Cube between the calf and hamstring, adjusting and/or repositioning to find new spots to treat. Choose to leave the toes tucked under or lay the top of the foot flat on the floor. If your knees can't handle this position, put a pillow or rolled up towel behind and/or under the knees.

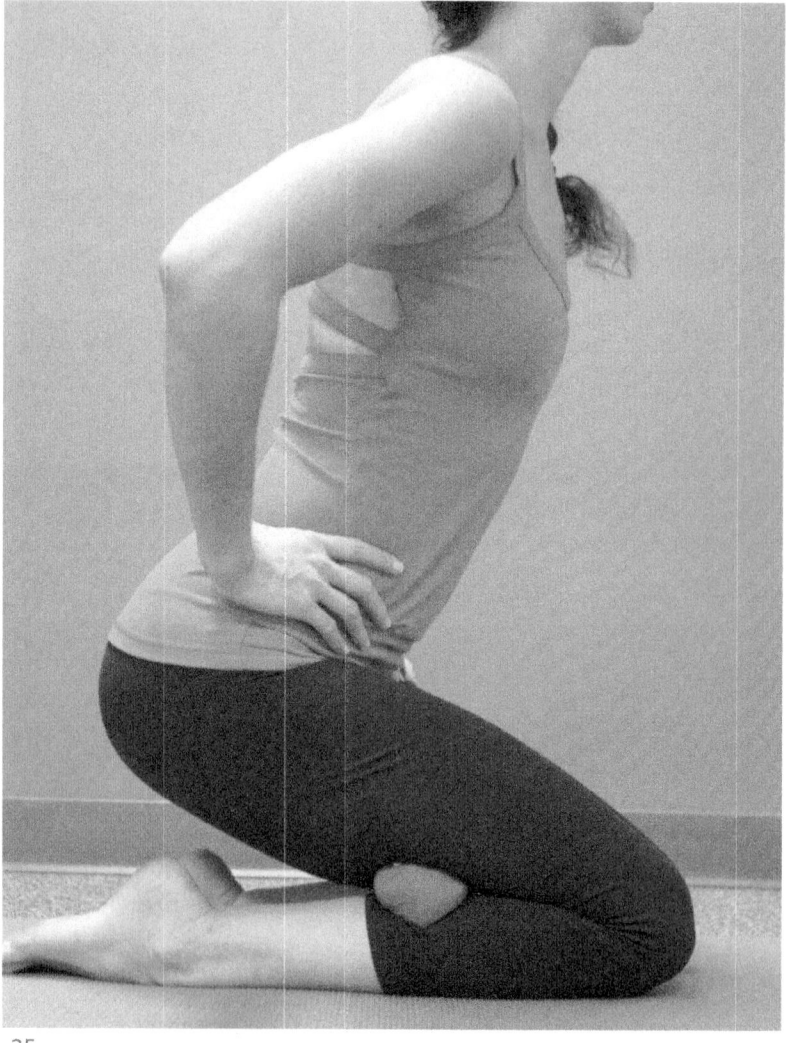

Re-test: Repeat the two tests below.

Look and feel for any calf, ankle, or Anterior Tibilalis tightness. You may notice improvement. That's great! You may notice a new areaof tightness that you can now address with the OMPT Cube™.

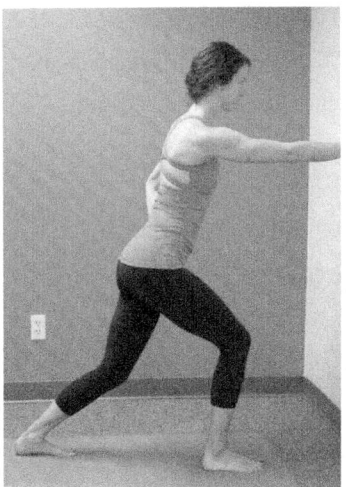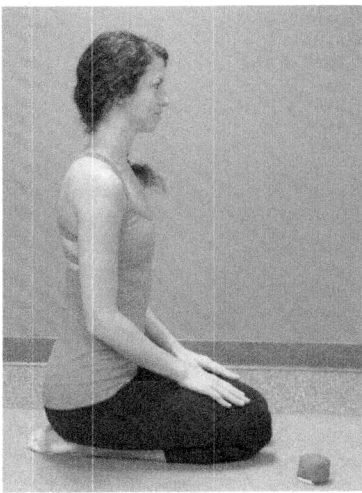

NOTE

Many people ask me how long they should use the omPT Cube in any one spot. There's no real right or wrong answer here. You get to listen to your body. After working on a specific area with the omPT Cube, you should feel a release or an improvement after a few minutes. If not, you may want to let it rest and revisit the area another time.

26

Spine and Hamstrings

Test: Staff pose.

Seated with legs long in front of you, lift up through the head, then hinge at the hips with a long spine. When you can hinge no further, round forward. Look and feel for spine or hamstring tightness.

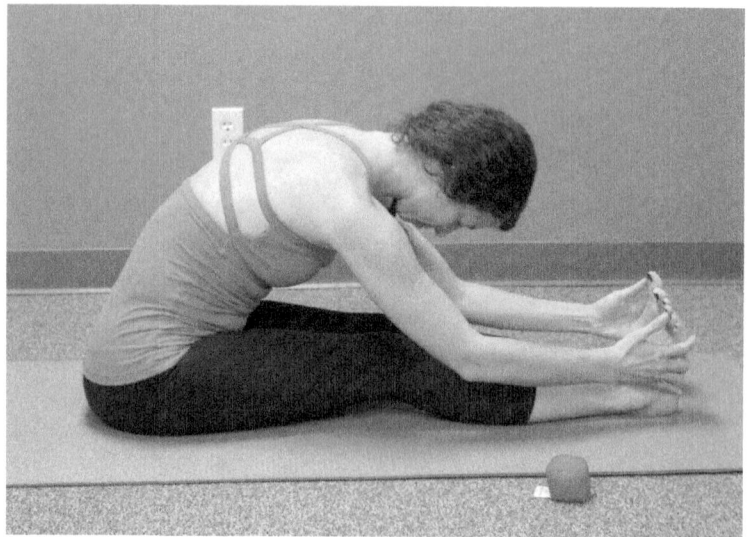

FUN FACT

Orthopedic Manual Physical Therapists, Chiropractors, and Osteopaths treat the mechanics of the spine using mobilization / manipulation. omPT Cube is a gentle way to support this type of bodywork.

Treat: Upper, mid, and lower spine.

Following either side of the bony landmarks of the spinous processes, use the omPT Cube to massage areas of tightness or tenderness. Include movement like a gentle rocking side to side. You may simply lay over the omPT Cube and feel the pressure increase as you take a full inhale and allow the torso to expand with your breath. Keep your feet planted on the floor with knees bent as a protective measure for the low back.

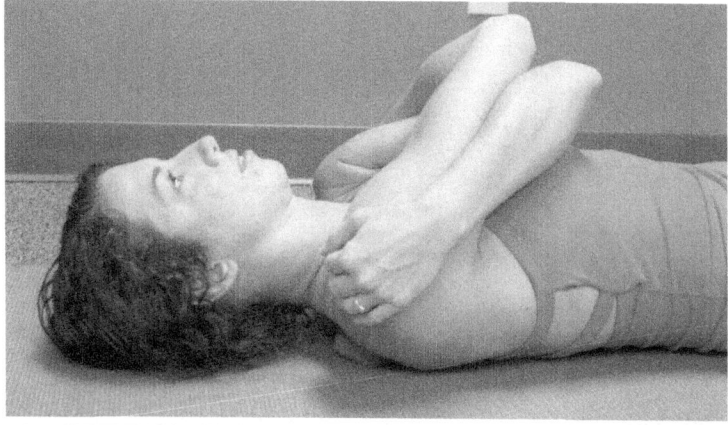

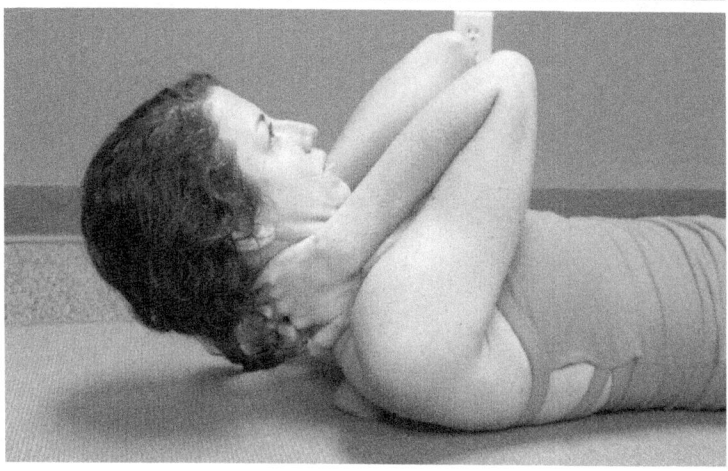

Treat (continued): Upper, mid, and lower spine.

Along the upper spine, you can increase pressure on the omPT Cube by crossing your arms over your chest or lifting the hips up while the feet remain planted.

Along the lower spine, increase pressure by drawing one or both knees toward your chest.

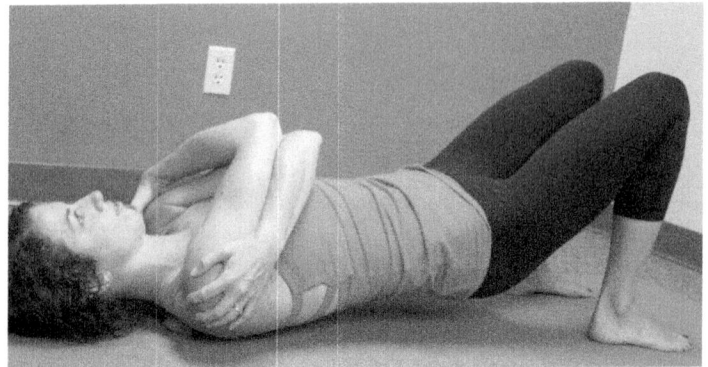

Treat: Hamstrings.

Sitting on the floor or in a chair, place the omPT Cube under your hamstrings. Sit tall through the spine, then with foot flexed, start to extend the leg. Move slowly and reposition the omPT Cube as needed.

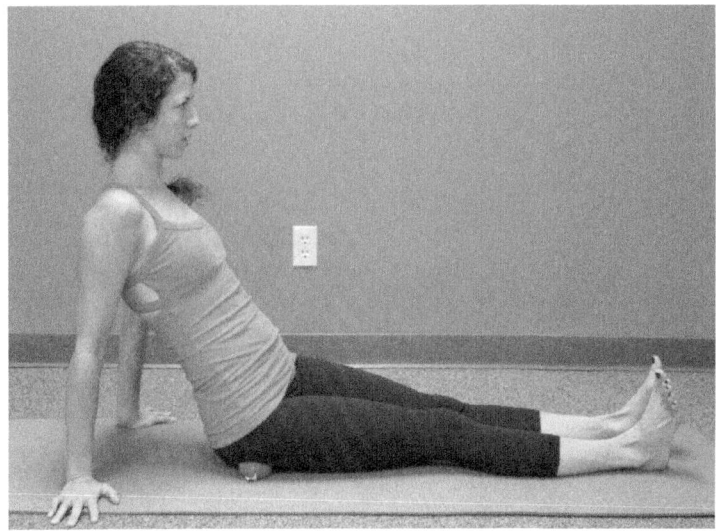

Re-test: Staff pose.

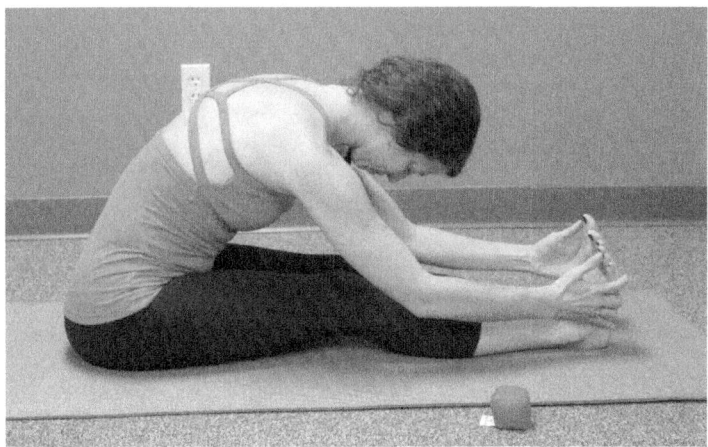

Movement: Adding bigger movements to your body care routine with omPT Cube helps to integrate the treatment of the muscles with a global approach to functional fitness.

Try any of the following movements for strengthening and stretching:

Child's pose

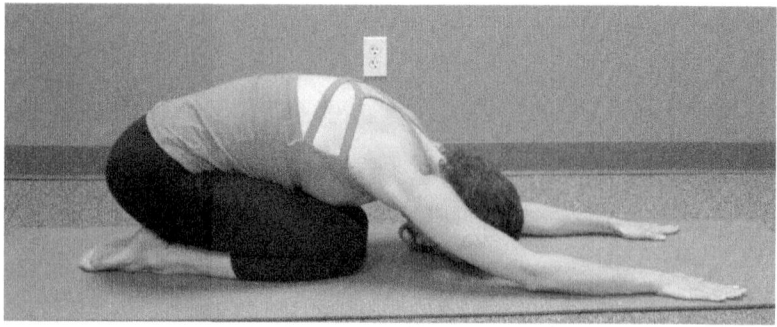

Child's pose with hands to one side, breathing into side body

Cat & Cow

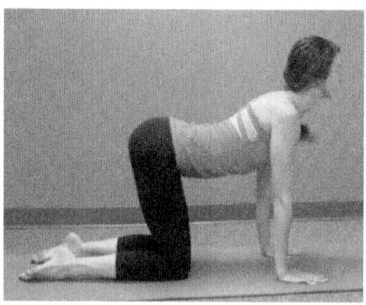 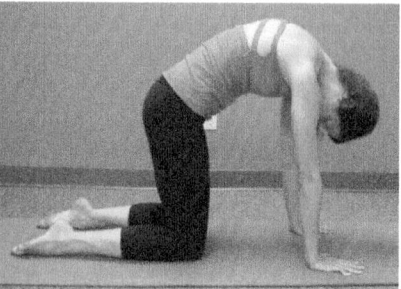

Cat & Cow with lateral bends side to side

x
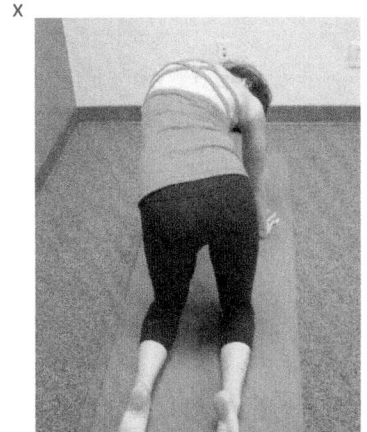
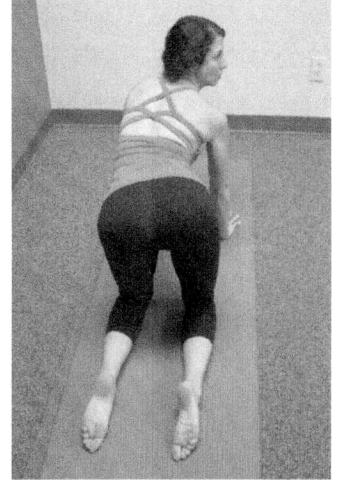

Down dog   Plank

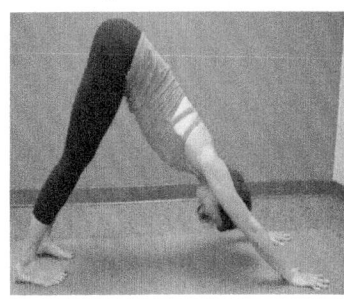
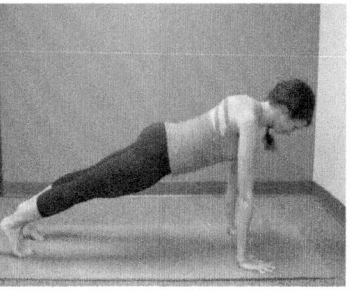

Up dog   Child's Pose

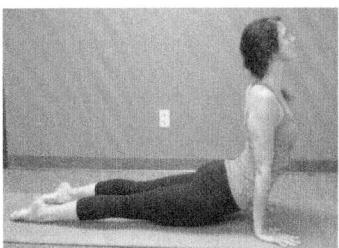
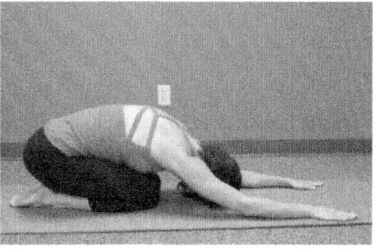

Hips

Test: Lie on your back and place one ankle above the opposite knee in a Figure Four position. Keep hips level. Look and feel for any areas of tightness or limited mobility. Then, bend the knee and bring toward the chest and across to the opposite shoulder. Again, look and feel for areas of tightness or limited mobility.

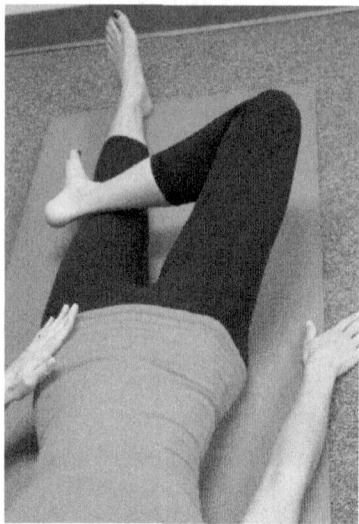 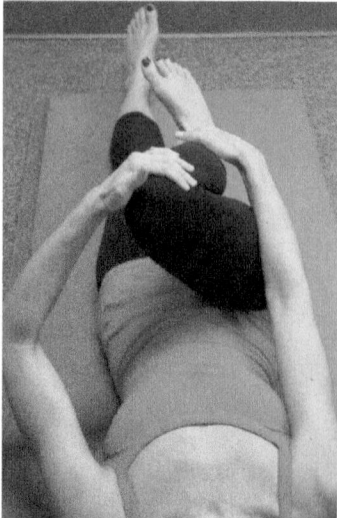

FUN FACT

The hips have the potential to hold deep emotions in the body. Are your hips particularly tight? Do you experience any release of emotion when stretching or using the omPT Cube on your hips?

Treat: Lower outer and inner hips.

Lying down, start by placing the omPT Cube under the area of your hips where you would put your hands in the back pockets of your pants. Move to the inner hips, finding the spot between your tailbone and sitz bone on either side. You may find better access to this area by sitting up on top of the omPT Cube.

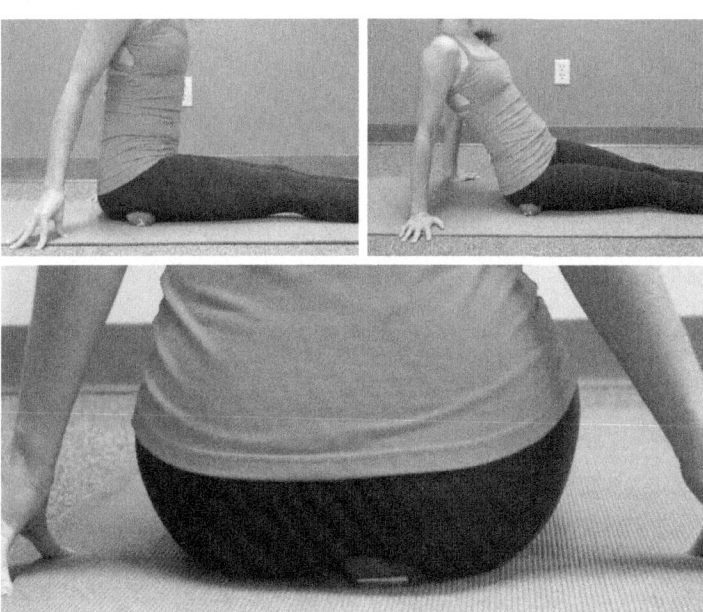

> **NOTE**
>
> Remember that you can use the omPT Cube in many different places and in many different ways. If you don't feel much in one spot, adjust the positioning of the omPT Cube and find a new spot. Keep breathing and explore different motions (360 degree movement).

Treat: Outer hips and front of hip.

Lying down, move the omPT Cube further to the outside of the hip. Begin to roll over on top of the omPT Cube to treat this area. Roll further onto the side of the body and place the omPT Cube along the front of the hip just below the bony landmark of your hip bone.

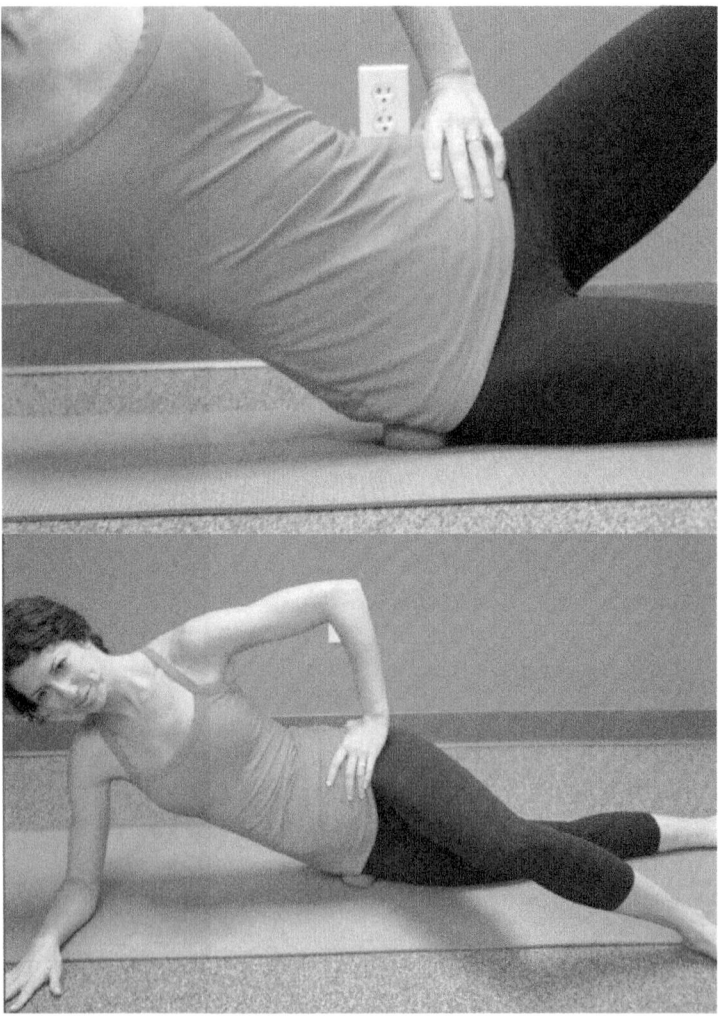

Re-test: Repeat the tests below.

Look and feel for any improvement in tightness or mobility.
Remember that you can treat any area again that still feels tight.

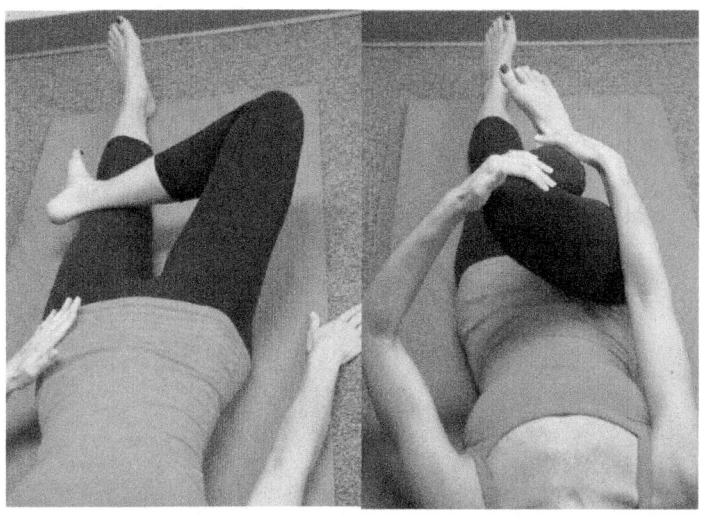

Movement:

Knee to Chest   Supine Cobbler's Pose

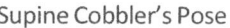

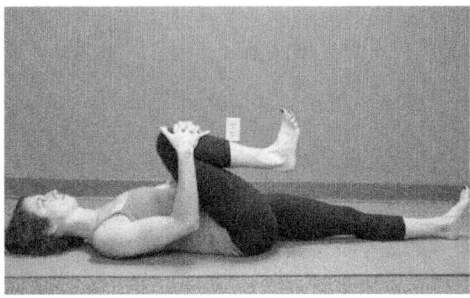
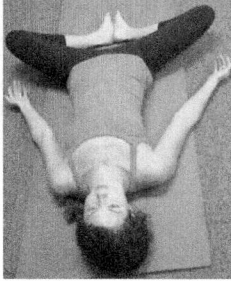

Movement (continued):

Reclined Half Pigeon

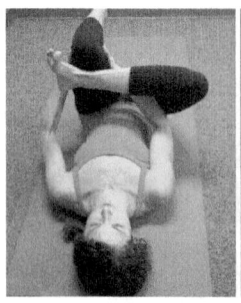 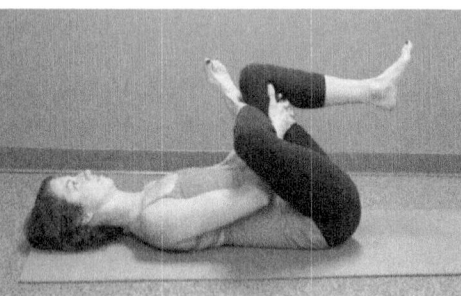

Half Pigeon

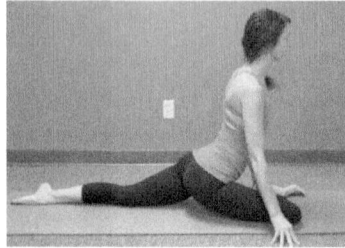 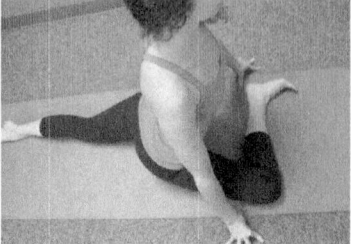

Frog - gently move forward and backward

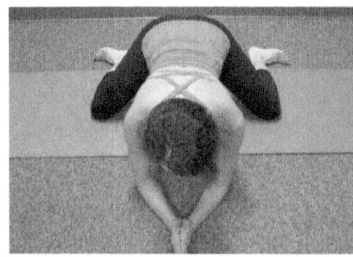 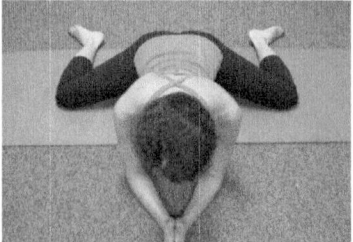

Child's pose

Shoulders & Upper Back

Test: Functional Shoulder Reach.

Sitting tall, reach the right arm overhead, bend at the elbow and slide the hand down the spine with the palm facing the back. The left hand reaches behind and up the spine with the palm facing out. Repeat on the other side. Look and feel for areas of tightness and any differences from side to side.

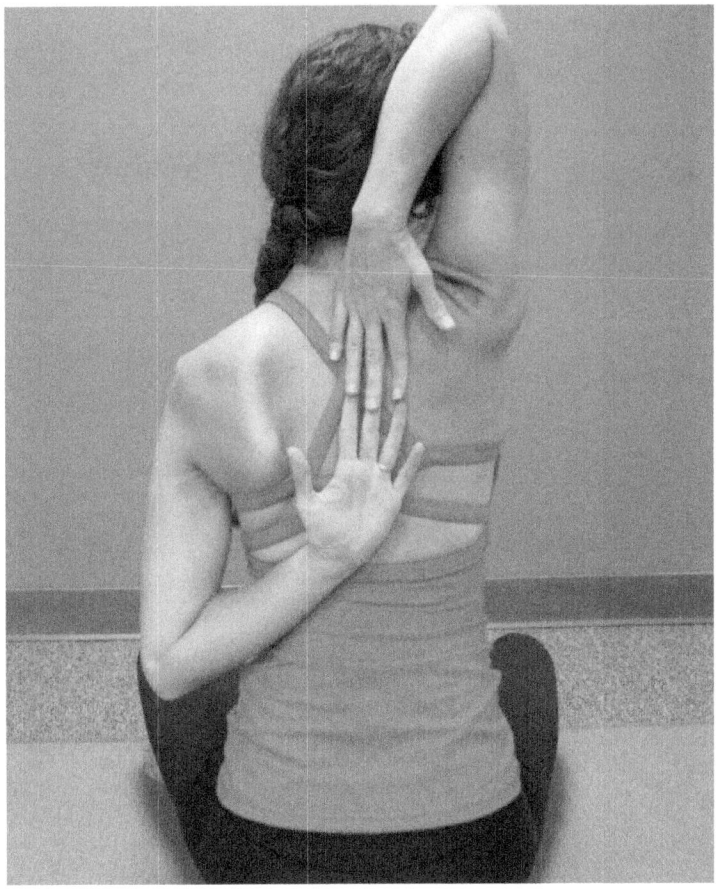

Treat: Front shoulder and chest.

Lying face down with arms extended to the side, place the omPT Cube under the pectoralis major and/or minor muscles on one side. Place the opposite hand under the shoulder and begin to roll back toward the extended arm.

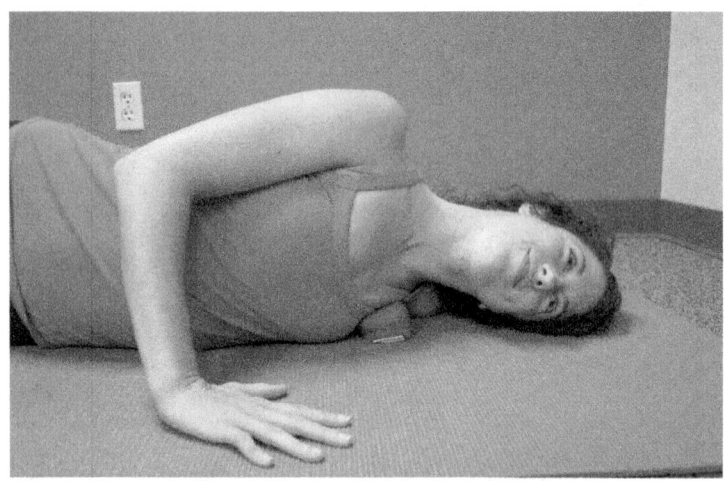

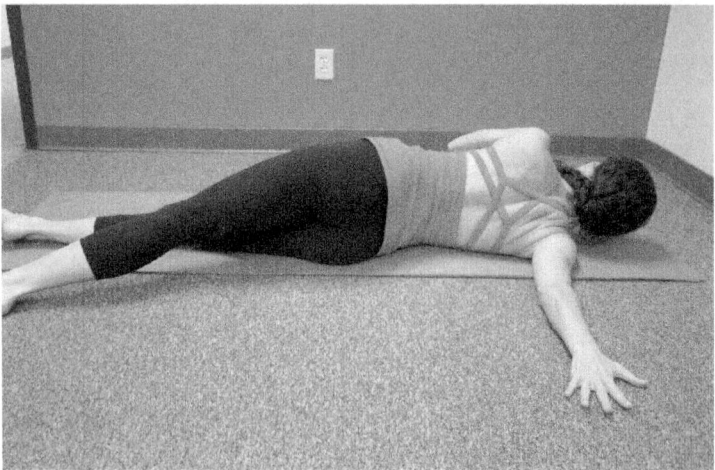

Gently change the angle of the shoulder and arm as desired. Then move the omPT Cube to the ball of the front of the shoulder and repeat the movement.

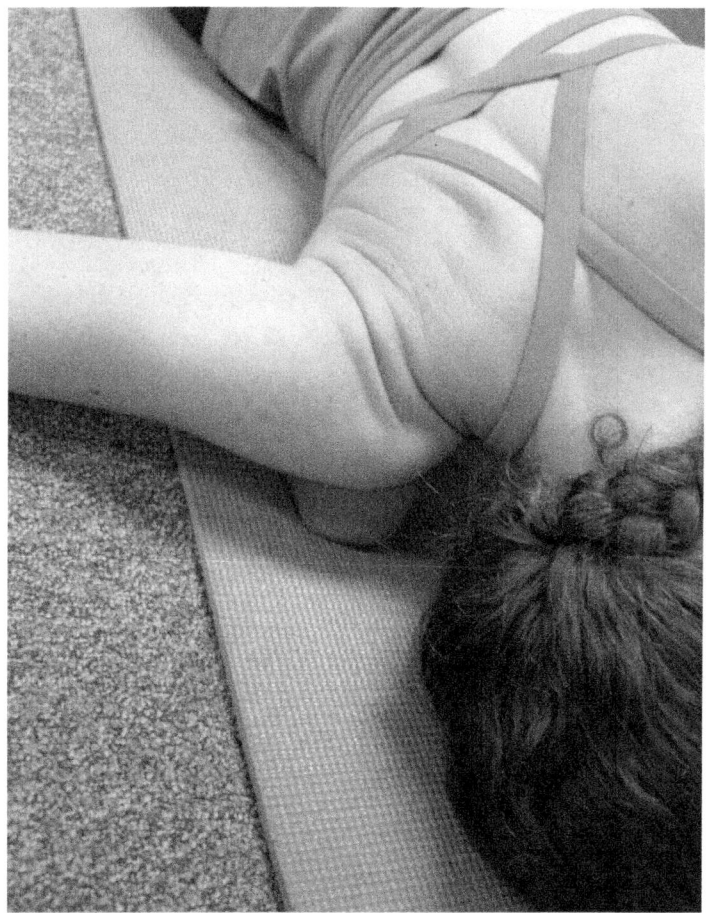

FUN FACT

"Forward Head Syndrome" and "Text Neck" describe similar conditions involving a flexed neck, rounded shoulders, and slumped upper back. Using the omPT Cube along the upper back can help improve your overall posture and reduce strain.

Re-test: Repeat the Functional Shoulder Reach side to side.

Also repeat the Staff Pose test here, as that position involves the full spine, hamstrings, as well as upper spine and shoulder carriage.

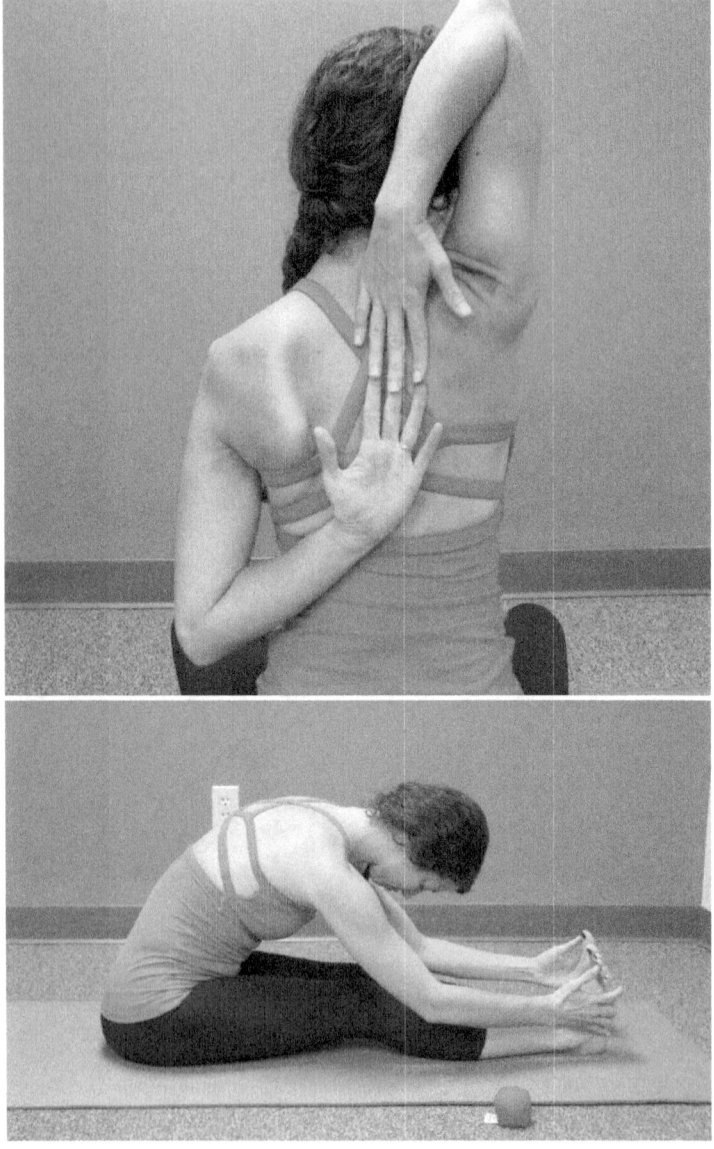

Movement:

Thread the Needle   Child's pose

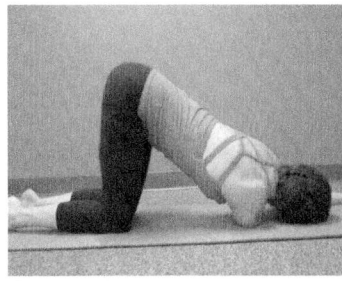 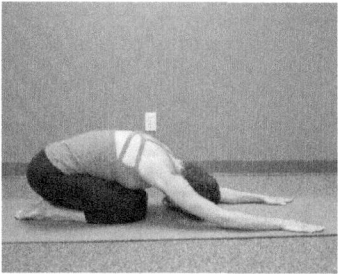

Rest – lie on your back and rest completely. Focus on breathing.

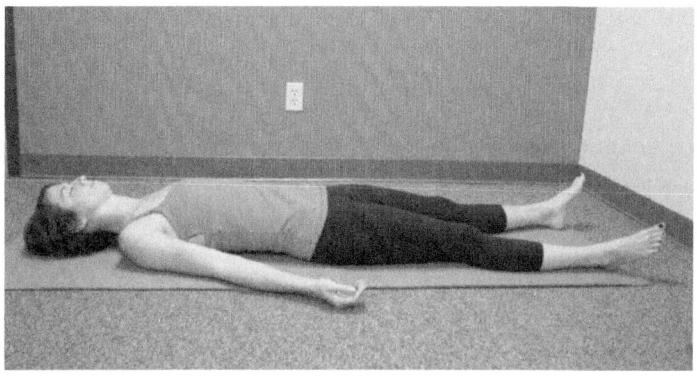

Where should the omPT Cube NOT be used?

As mentioned before, the omPT Cube can be used anywhere there is muscle. There are certain areas of the body in particular you'll want to avoid, namely bony areas and vascular tissue. Use this chart as a guide.

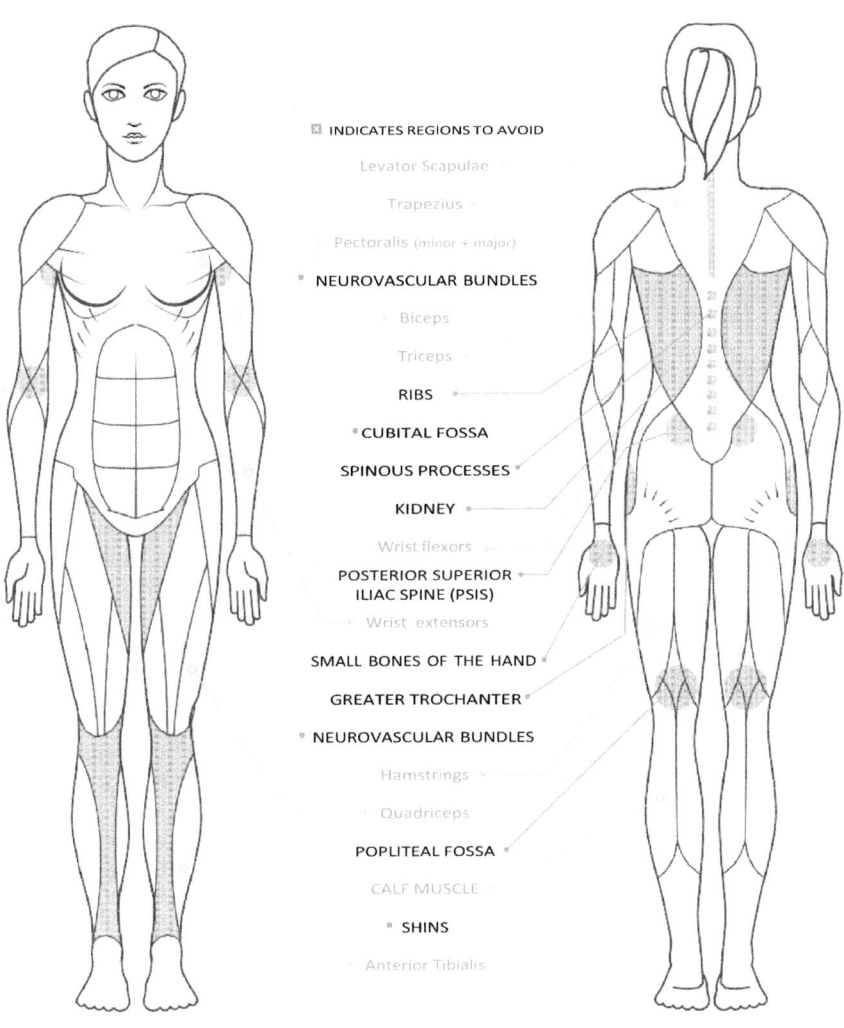

⊠ INDICATES REGIONS TO AVOID

Levator Scapulae

Trapezius

Pectoralis (minor + major)

NEUROVASCULAR BUNDLES

Biceps

Triceps

RIBS

CUBITAL FOSSA

SPINOUS PROCESSES

KIDNEY

Wrist flexors

POSTERIOR SUPERIOR
ILIAC SPINE (PSIS)

Wrist extensors

SMALL BONES OF THE HAND

GREATER TROCHANTER

NEUROVASCULAR BUNDLES

Hamstrings

Quadriceps

POPLITEAL FOSSA

CALF MUSCLE

SHINS

Anterior Tibialis

The Program

If you have 5-15 minutes available, pick any area(s) of the body to treat. If you have small amounts of time available throughout the day, you may be able to address the whole body!

If you have 20 minutes or more, begin with the feet and work your way up the entire body. Personalize the experience based on what you're feeling in your body, taking more time or less in different areas.

If you have one hour or more, consider using one of the following Whole Body omPT Cube plans.

Whole Body
omPT Cube Plans

Activity		60-min	90-min
Lower legs		13 min	20 min
Test Calves		1 min	2 min
Treat Feet		1 min each	21/2 min each
Test ankle in heel sitting		1 min	1 min
Treat Anterior Shin / Ankles		2 min each	21/2 min each
Treat Calves		2 min each	21/2 min each
Re-test Calves + Anterior Shin / Ankle		1 min	2 min
Spine		16 min	25 min
Test Staff pose		1 min	11/2 min
Treat Spine	Base of neck / upper back	1 min each	2 min each
	Thoracic Spine	11/2 min each	2 min each
	Lumbar Spine	11/2 min each	2 min each
	Sacrum	1 min each	2 min each
Re-test Staff pose		1 min	1 1/2 min
Choose Movement	Child's pose	4 min flow	6 min flow
	Cat / Cow		
	Thread the needle, with arm up		
	Down dog, with leg up		
	Plank		
	Chatarunga		
	Up dog		
	Child's pose		

Activity (continued)			
Hips		13 min	20 min
Test Hips		1 min	2 min
Treat Hips	Gluteus Medius	11/2 min each	2 min each
	Rotators	11/2 min each	2 min each
	Inner Hip	1 min each	2 min each
	Outside Hip	1/2 min each	1/2 min each
Re-test Hips		1 min	1 min
Choose Movement	Knee to chest	2 min flow	4 min flow
	Supine Cobbler's Pose		
	Reclined Half Pigeon		
	Frog – gently move forward and backward		
	Child's pose		
Shoulder Girdle		13 min	20 min
Test Functional Reach		1 min	1 min
Test Shoulder Girdle	Anterior Shoulder	11/2 min each	2 min each
	Back of Shoulder Blade	11/2 each	2 min each
	Sides of Shoulder Blade	1 min each	2 min each
Re-test	Functional Shoulder Reach	1 min	1 min
	Staff Pose - Seated Forward Bend	1 min	1 min
Choose Movement	Child's pose	2 min	5 min
	Shavasana		

What now?

1. Consistency! The omPT Cube only works if you use it. This is where we get to partner. We're Better Together! Find a routine that works for you and do your best to remain consistent.

2. Share the omPT Cube with someone else so we can heal the world together. Consider creating a group that meetsregularly to use the OMPT Cube together.

3. Bodyworkers and fitness professionals can get trained in omPT Cube workshops and instruction as a therapist or trainer. It is a great way to diversify your offerings and increase your income.

See www.RebeccaLowe.physio for more information.

BONUS Guided Meditation

For best results, self-treatment and self-care involves all aspects of our being and encompasses not just our body, but our heart, mind, and spirit as well.

The omPT Cube as it's laid out here focuses mostly on the physical body, but there are ways to bring the other parts of us to the work we are doing for our body. You are a whole person and all parts are inter-connected.

Here are some concepts that can help us connect to all of us:

Body

The body is always, always on our side. It is always trying to help us. Does our body know that we are on its side? Does it know we will care for it? Have we been caring for our body? The omPT Cube is one way. Are there other ways we need to start caring for our body?

The body is a truth-teller and it is trying to communicate with us. Can we hear what it is saying? Sometimes it is whispering, sometimes talking, and sometimes yelling. Are we listening? Sometimes it is telling us to modify or stop a certain activity or change our ergonomics. Sometimes the body is telling us something about a relational or emotional story. Is there an association with pain or tension in your body and a relationship or situation that is causing it or making it worse?

You can trust your body. It will tell you what you need. And it will tell you where and how long to work on each spot.

Emotion

The body is holding so much for us. We hold stress and emotions in our body. And we hold them in specific places. Can we tell what emotion or stress we are storing where?

As we are working on our body, is there anything we can let go of? Is it time? Are we in a safe place and can now let go of the tension and emotion that we've been holding there? While we are working on our body, we can sometimes identify what we need to work on in our life as well.

Mind

Our minds can run us in circles. How aware are we of our thoughts, negative loops, or distractions? Sometimes we are doing so much cognitive management that we never really get to rest. If you notice your brain doing this, you most likely need to do some work in the conscious and subconscious realms. But, for now, there is benefit in allowing your mind and body to rest. See if you can allow your thoughts to flow through while practicing the omPT Cube .

Spirit

The deepest part of us holds our beliefs. What we believe significantly affects our life, emotions, thoughts, and body.

Do I know where I am in the world?

Is the world a safe place?

Is there Something higher than me?

Is that a benevolent and loving Something?

Is everything on my shoulders?

Do I believe something about my body that isn't allowing me to change my story?

Can I heal?

Am I valuable?

Is everything something I have to fight for or can I rest when needed?

Do I have control over my life?

Do I have help and support from those around me?

I have included a Listening Meditation Practice that may help you connect to Love and to yourself. I encourage you to integrate all parts of yourself. It is worth it. You are worth it. You can become your authentic self in the world, get rid of negative loops or patterns, and change your story.

BONUS Listening Meditation

(Body, Mind, Heart, and Spirit)

Go through this process as often as you need to connect to yourself (body, mind, heart, spirit) and to Spirit.

It can bring up powerful emotions, so take your time. There is no rush. All of it is good and part of the process. Listen to yourself. If needed, reach out to someone that is safe and can be there with you or help you through the beginning of this type of inner work. Often, after you learn how to process this way, you can do it yourself.

I will be using various faith words that you can choose to leave out of your practice entirely, or substitute with the term that you connect to. For instance, if God or Spirit is not what you use, but you use Universe, Energy, Light, or Love, then use that. They are interchangeable as long as what you connect to is a feeling of safety, Love, and Presence.

Find a quiet place where you will not be disturbed. Try to set aside at least 20 minutes. You can sit or lie down. You may journal as you go, or write what you hear later.

1. Notice how your body is feeling.

Do you have tightness anywhere? Is your breathing constricted? What do you think of your breathing? Are you feeling anxious? Angry? Do you have pain anywhere?

2. Notice your surroundings.

What sounds do you hear? Is anyone around you? Can you hear them breathing or sighing? Are there any birds nearby or crickets? The wind? Street noises or lawnmowers? Can you feel the wind or the sun on your face? Are you sitting on a hard surface, a cushion, or a mat? Can you feel anything else? Someone else's energy?

3. Now, try to let all of that pass through your mind.

Let it go for now. If a thought comes through about dinner tonight, or you left your wash in the washer, or something with work, or kids, let it drift on by. Each time it happens during your meditation, let those details of life thoughts pass on by, becoming distant for now. You'll come back to it later. It will wait for you.

4. Breathe in and out for several minutes.

Slow your breath down and focus on matching the breath in and out. Aim for 5 seconds in, 5 seconds out. Try to control it so that it takes 5 seconds to fully inspire and then by the end of 5 seconds you have gotten rid of all of your air. Allow yourself to breathe so that you breathe into all directions equally – front, back, sides, down, up.

5. Mentally picture and feel a time where you have felt completely safe and loved.

It may be a memory, or a physical place that you have been, or just a feeling. If that feeling is associated with Spirit or Love, go ahead and imagine being connected. Imagine that that feeling of Love and safety and acceptance has something to give to you right now. Open yourself to receiving whatever Love wants to give to you. Feel what it feels like to be completely loved. Feel how you don't have to work or strive for it. There is nothing you have to do to be more loved than you are right now. You are already completely loved and accepted.

6. Say the first gratitude that comes to mind.

"Thank you for ..."

7. Here is a prayer that you can pray if you are comfortable with the words and concepts:

Spirit, I know You are with me and in me. You have always been with me. I know you are with me now. Thank you.

I pray for protection over me and this place and the universe around me – every- where I go, everywhere I am, and over everyone I have authority to pray this. Lift off oppression from those that are oppressed. Give hope and joy. Remove any negative spirituality, curses, unhealthy intentions, and hooks. Remove negative loops. And help me change wrong beliefs about myself, you, people, and the world. Heal trauma and memories down to the cellular level.

Show me who I am – show me your beautiful and true view of me. Show me how I was made originally. Help me identify where I am still holding pain and what part of me is having to do this. Please help that part of me know that they can rest and that they do not need to do that anymore by themselves. All parts of me are acceptable and can all function together. Nothing needs to be fractured anymore. I am whole. Give me insight and direction. Help me stop striving and performing for others. Help me to truly rest. Help me to hear and to trust myself.

8. Choose one of the following four options for med-itation and listening today:

Just rest and let go of striving.

Re-connect with Presence and go into a mode of receiving. Receive whatever God has for you today. You do not have to do anything to receive it. You are valuable and you just need to be you. And today, you just need to rest and receive. Make sure you are breathing deeply and slowly. And keep receiving. See if you can feel safe and feel connected.

Read a passage from a wisdom book.

Read until you find something that speaks directly to you or resonates in your soul. Meditate on it. Read it over several times. Write it down in a journal if you like.   And then, go into a listening mode. What do you hear?

Listening to the part of us that is holding pain, either emotional or physical.

Start to "look" for that part of you that is needing you to under-stand them. It may be the part of you that is hurting right now. Often, the part of you that has been holding pain usually feels alone. You have had to fracture off that part of you because it was too painful and you had to isolate it to be able to function. It may be the part of you that needs to sleep a lot, or watch movies all the time, or use a substance to cover up pain, or has to be funny all the time.

See if you can connect to that part of you, maybe even visualize what that part of you looks like – it may be male or female, or young or old, look like a teacher you had, or a parent.

Or listen to anything you hear about yourself. If the voice you hear is critical or mean, then that is not Spirit or Love, that may be a part of you that has had to be critical. It may be saying, that "This is ridiculous. This can't help you. You can't hear anything." You can go ahead and identify and talk to that part of you. It's a part of you that you have needed. It has been helping you. You do not want to get rid of any part of you, only be able to hear and understand and bring all parts of you together, so they don't have to be alone.

At this point you may hear any number of things. There is no pattern and no right answer. If you don't hear anything or visualize anything, that is okay. Just allow yourself to focus on breathing right now and staying in the place that feels safe.

If you do hear or visualize anything, then make sure there is no shame, or judgement, or fear associated with it. Just be present with yourself.

Can you visualize being able to get rid of the pain that part of you has been holding? How would you like to get rid of it? Will someone take it away? Can you burn it? Flush it down a toilet? Whatever you do, try to let it go. If it is a physical sensation, then imagine being able to let it go, breathe it out, have it seep out of you. Try to unbrace anywhere that you feel braced.

Now talk to that part of you that has been holding the pain. Let them know that they have done a really, really good job. They have held so much for perhaps a really long time. They do not have to hold it alone anymore. They have been needed and still are needed, but they don't need to function all alone anymore. They will know when they need to do their job, but now together.

If there is sadness and grief, or anger, or whatever emotion comes up through this process, it is all good and fine. Let it all out, for as long as it needs to come out. It may have been locked up for a long time. Feel it all. Bring your presence and Loving Presence to it. You are not alone, even if you thought you were. All parts of you are there and Love is there. You never have to feel alone again.

Questions and Directions.

Go into the same place with trying to hear from different parts of you and from Love, but this time bring whatever question you want to ask yourself. Perhaps a question on something about who you are or a life question. Just listen without judgement to what you hear. You may hear different perspectives. Then you can ask further questions like, what part of me is saying that? Is it the wise or fearful part of me? Is that the little child? Is that the part that dreams?

9. You can write things down that you have heard.

You have done great internal work and it will already have shifted things. Re-connect with your body and see if there have been any changes in body sensations – tension, pain, lightness, breathing, …

10. You can end with this prayer:

To Love, thank you for being with me and helping me see and hear and feel what I needed to today. Thank you for allowing a change in what needed to shift today within my heart, body, mind, spirit including subconscious and negative memories that may have been held in my body. Allow more movement, freedom, and joy. Allow me to feel your Love in abundance.

11. You can use this meditation along with using the omPT Cube.

Letting things go emotionally and physically at the same time. Or, listening to your body's wisdom as you work on yourself.

Elements of this meditation and listening practice are influenced by Cynthia Bourgeault, Andrew Miller, and Mark Virkler. For further exploration into internal work and centering prayer, you can look for further resources by these authors and teachers.

THE omPT CUBE:

A tool to empower you to heal through the combined knowledge and practice of yoga and PT

Made in the USA
Middletown, DE
01 August 2022

70310625R00040